e-Mental Health: Progress, Challenge, and Change

Edited by:
Austin Mardon, Catherine Mardon

Written by:
John Christy Johnson, Peter Anto Johnson,
Shawna Harline, Robert McWeeny

Copyright © 2021 by Austin Mardon
All rights reserved. This book or any portion thereof may not be reproduced or used in any manner whatsoever without the express written permission of the publisher except for the use of brief quotations in a book review or scholarly journal.

First Printing: 2021

Typeset and Cover Design by Justine Nicole Banszky

ISBN 978-1-716-25136-8

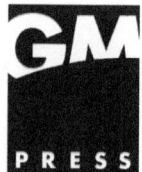

Golden Meteorite Press
103 11919 82 St NW
Edmonton, AB T5B 2W3
www.goldenmeteoritepress.com

Dedicated to everyone around the globe whose mental health has been affected, particularly those suffering from the repercussions of the COVID-19 pandemic.

4.	1. Introduction
6.	2. E-mental Health and Autonomy
15.	3. Adverse Physical and Psychological Health Effects
23.	4. Cyberwars and e-mental health: whatearn from the past?
30.	5. E-mental Health Tool: Clinical VR
41.	6. The Future of Mental Health in the Era of COVID-19
52.	7. Digitizing Information
66.	8. Stigma
81.	9. Kids & Mobile Apps: Generational gaps
87.	10. Conclusion

1. INTRODUCTION

What is e-mental health? Perhaps the most common usage of the phrase stems from the many services online that aim to deliver mental health information, resources, and support through the Internet, apps, videoconferencing, virtual reality, and other technology. However, we recognize this phrase as far more expansive and broad. When we break it down, the prefix e- indicates electronic and mental health refers to our psychological well-being. When combined, we draw the expansive definition for e-mental health: our psychological well-being in an electronic space. This electronic space can be any aspect of the digital world - virtual reality, social media, entertainment, apps, websites, etc.

Preserving one's mental health in a digital world is more than a challenge for many, especially our youth. A striking 60% of teens report some form of bullying or harassment online and over 90% concede it is one of the predominant and concerning problems within their age category. Targets of cyberbullying and stress online are at a greater risk for self-harm and suicidal behaviour. A worrying 18% of youth report engaging in self-harming behaviour at least once and a still disturbing 6% admit to digitally harming themselves or others through anonymous posts and/or sharing content about themselves. Coupled with these statistics, approximately 10% of the general population experience digital addictions - whether this be addictions to gambling, shopping, pornography, games, social media, or some other form of entertainment. Not only are many of these habits unhealthy in promoting a sedentary lifestyle for us, they can also bring about adverse effects neurologically and lead to negative thoughts about loneliness, isolation, and a lack of connection to reality.

    Nonetheless, the fact is that several elements of the digital world also come with much benefits to mental health. With almost half of the world using the internet today, we also recognize that several of these activities allow individuals to be productive, to destress and find refuge from stressful lifestyles, or find a safe space to connect with others. It has enabled financial stability for many and soon, half of jobs are projected to be online over the next decade. Many applications such as virtual care even enable us to promote mental health through resources, counseling, therapies, and the use of artificial intelligence. Perhaps the very dual nature of the digital world and its uncertain effects on our mental health is precisely what makes it worth exploring deeper. This book has aimed to explore these mysterious effects on mental health, how we have observed them over the years, and what we can expect for the future.

2. E-mental Health and Autonomy

How many times have we checked the "I have read all terms and conditions" without reading the terms and conditions? When it comes down to it, how do we ensure that our autonomy is protected in the digital world? The freedom to live the way we want to in the digital world is perhaps similar to our rights and freedoms in the physical world. There are laws in the physical world which are enforceable are strengthened by social norms and law enforcement, whereas laws of cyberspace are more difficult to enforce. Most notably, multiple forms of internet addictions develop quite easily due to the accessibility and anonymity offered by the net. For example, entertainment, social media, pornography, gambling, or even online shopping and retail are among common addictions that can develop, perhaps all the more easily when one's anonymity is protected. Nonetheless, the designs to ensure security and privacy online are undoubtedly necessary to protect highly sensitive or confidential information about identity, finances, and other important personal information.

When we consider mental health in the digital world, many of the ethical principles applied in healthcare still apply. It may have once been a common understanding that the respect for autonomy and justice as a reactionary move to prevent exploitation by medical professionals, as was popularized by mass media and popular culture. Historically, medical ethics have reflected paternalistic tendencies specifically designed to "underpin the massive responsibility that fell on the shoulders of doctors," thereby overlooking patient autonomy as a whole in the physician-patient relationship (Williams & Kaley). Paternalism essentially eliminates patient agency by placing a greater degree of faith in the physician's expertise. In the modern age, there has been a dramatic shift towards treatment pathways centred around respect for patient autonomy instead. In the context of e-mental health, we must not only consider autonomy, we must also accommodate the priorities and goals of the individual, changes in psychological states of well-being, resource limitations in delivery of care or intervention, and technological limitations in this delivery for those with reduced mental capacities or altered mental states.

The unconscious mind can be easily influenced by the activities we engage in on the digital world, perhaps more so than in the physical world. In her book Better off Dead, Sarah Conly discusses paternalism and the persistent unconsciousness. We can examine her arguments on medical assistance in dying to gain insights into how we must respond to autonomy in the context of e-mental health. The case of dementia is often considered and very well one of the most controversial topics when we are discussing the changes in the level of an individual's autonomy. Conly champions a very extreme notion that we should "[kill] off helpless people who do no harm" particularly those who are in persistent vegetative states (PVS), bringing up this consideration of autonomy for patients requiring e-mental health care. In their article on advance directives, dementia, and physician-assisted death, Paul Menzel and Bonnie Steinbock develop the notion that the moral precedence of an advance directive, in the context of healthcare provided for individuals with dementia, should correlate with the extent to which it is grounded in information, thought, and fact. These two texts represent dual sides of a spectrum. Here, we examine to what degree respect for autonomy should play a role in creating decisions about e-mental health delivery and support offered for individuals with severe dementia with respect to the views of Conly and Menzel and Steinbock. This can be best done by contrasting Conly's paternalism approach to the autonomy-based approach championed by Menzel and Steinbock.

Let us consider the contemporary era, where paternalism has widespread negative connotations. Both online and in the physical world, environments where an autonomous entity controls our actions consciously can be created. The U.S. Public Health Service Study at Tuskegee explicitly highlights this point, in which doctors intentionally withheld penicillin from black men to study syphilis progression. Conly's blunt rebuttal effectively dispels a significant amount of 'fluff' or superfluous sentiment surrounding the glamorization of respect for autonomy as the be-all-end-all of medical ethics. Even in the scenario of severe dementia, Conly's points remain highly valid. Comparable to PVS, severe dementia incurs a significant cost to society. A RAND Corporation study in the United States revealed that the total monetary cost of dementia ranged from $157 to $215 billion per annum, rendering the disease more economically beleaguering than heart disease and cancer. While these numbers include dementia care in its less severe forms, from a resource-based view, it becomes apparent that dementia care is neither a cost-effective or time-efficient practice for healthcare providers, begging the question whether certain provisions for patient autonomy such as advance directives should be valued altogether. In the online sphere as well, we must consider the many inhibitions created by dependence, addictions, fatigue, and other conditions created by prolonged exposure to the digital environment that forces individuals to make decisions that may not be in their control. With a high global prevalence of up to 10% reported for internet addiction disorders and its associated neurological complications, psychological disturbances, and social problems, many of the costs match numbers indicating costs of dementia in our society. More concerning is the number of cases that go unreported or unnoticed given the fact it is not easy for an individual to recognize, admit, or even be aware of. People around these individuals may also have a difficult time discerning these symptoms. Similar to the authority figures and physicians of the Tuskegee experiments, marketers and online brands become motivated by the desire for profit through ads and traffic rather than the amount of time a potential consumer is spending time on their website.

Regardless of the ethical fabric of Menzel and Steinbock's claim, presenting patients or consumers with an autonomous choice for their care or health in consumption may demand an excessive societal burden for others. Furthermore, in most severe forms of dementia, recovery to a mentally competent state may practically be non-existent - quite similar to how addictions can progress to a point where individuals become blinded from their realities. This not only reiterates the wasteful nature of investing in continued support for those suffering from dementia but also beckons the question of whether providing supports through telehealthcare or virtual care for addictions and e-mental health problems, especially in light of COVID-19, truly reflects the best interest of the patient or whether it may be counterproductive. Conly's assertion that there is no benefit to the individual to keep them in a permanently unconscious state may be applied to these individuals as well. Note that in "severe" dementia, one is unable to speak daily more than 5-6 words, and may lack the ability to walk, sit up, hold up one's head, or smile. We observe similar signs in young peoples facing various drug addictions. As such, it can plausibly impair a severe dementic or person with altered mental health, due to their overexposure to the virtual world, and their capacity to participate or possess characteristically human qualities (experience, autonomy, goal completion, etc.).

 Intimately interconnected with this idea is Conly's condemnation of advance directives for treatment as "a result of poor reasoning." While recovery from dementia is not as popularized in mass media as patient awaking from comas, patients (in their competent state of writing the advance directive) and families may still be blinded by heuristics and hope of recovery that inhibit them from making a rational decision. Now consider this in the arena of e-mental health: how can we know when a severe addict has recovered or what phase of his progression he is in? Conly may suggest that there is no way to tell and as a result, relying on their judgment at any point in time may be meaningless.

But let us extend this notion even further. From a biological view, causes of dementia are typically permanent, comprising of deposition of plaques, neurofibrillary tangles, or blood vessel abnormalities. As such, there is a psychological discontinuity dividing the individual's primary interests before and following neurodegeneration. A person who has an internet addiction disorder, for instance, faces similar changes physiologically to those who have drug addictions. The brain's volume decreases and both white and grey matter shrinks leading to loss of primary interests, emotional processing, and brain functioning. Menzel and Steinbock refer to Dworkin's dichotomy of critical and experiential interests to better illustrate these critical interests. In summary, critical interests, a characteristic largely attributed to the individual's psychological state prior to disease progression, are second-order values that require careful deliberation and evaluation while experiential interests refers to the first-order notion of basic desire that are attributed more so with the human experience. In contrast to Conly's views on the futility of advanced directives or decision-making capacities of individuals, Menzel and Steinback suggest advanced directives are designed to circumvent the problem of these individuals' incapacity to uphold their own autonomy. This suggests individuals who have not progressed to severe addiction states can be identified and helped. Note that situations in which patients are intermediately demented are still excluded from this category, as the natures of the decisions created become more susceptible to the whims of the disease. Following dementia progression, the capacity to form new critical interests decreases. The fundamental conflict arises when experiential interests clash with the critical interests represented in advance directives.

Then how should we determine when the autonomy of an individual takes priority. Take for example, the case of former nurse Margot Bentley, an 83-year-old Alzheimer's patient in her final stage, who signed an advance directive stating, "she should be allowed to die if she suffered from an extreme disability with no expectation of recovery." Despite this, the care home provided her with proper nourishment. The family challenged the health care providers in court for spoon-feeding her without consent, thereby constituting battery. In this case, the court ruled against this, deeming that "Ms. Bentley was capable of making the decision to open her mouth and be fed, and the spoon-feeding constituted personal care rather than health care." The court may value this "decision" as one centred in Ms. Bentley's experiential interests and her autonomy in the here and now as opposed to the personal directive relayed from her 'past self.' However, Menzel and Steinbock would concur with the family to respect the patient's advance directive as "who she [had] become [was] not who she was when she wrote her living will." According to her family, Ms. Bentley had verbally explained her intentions to them and the most respectful course of action would have been to comply with the advance directive. But how would we measure these parameters in light of e-mental health, where such agreements may not exist? How would we judge that an individual with a mental health problem is suffering or being cared for?

Taken collectively, we need to recognize that autonomy should play a limited role in creating decisions about healthcare delivery and support offered for individuals with severe addictions. As indicated by Conly, the time, effort, and cost associated with care are wasteful in nature and as suggested through Menzel and Steinbock, seeking to respect autonomy is fraught with skirmishes between experiential and critical interests. Ultimately, these are both sides to consider when e-mental health is being considered.

References
Williams SJ, Caley L. Improving Healthcare Services: Co-production, Codesign and Operations [Internet]. Springer International Publishing; 2020. Available from: https://books.google.ca/books?id=iTfSDwAAQBAJ

Conly, Sarah. Better Off Dead. 2016. "Paternalism and Persistent Unconsciousness." p. 287-295.

Menzel, Paul T. and Steinbock, Bonnie. Journal of Law, Medicine, and Ethics. 2013. "Advance Directives, Dementia, and Physician-Assisted Death"

Hamblin, James. "The Doctor Used to Know Best." The Atlantic. May 19, 2014. Accessed December 07, 2020.

https://www.theatlantic.com/health/archive/2014/05/the-doctor-used-to-know-best/371170/).

Hurd, Michael D., Paco Martorell, Adeline Delavande, Kathleen J. Mullen, and Kenneth M. Langa. "Cost of Dementia Tops $159 Billion Annually in the United States." RAND Corporation. April 01, 2013. Accessed December 09, 2017. https://www.rand.org/pubs/external_publications/EP50247.html.

"Can You Recover From Dementia?" The Memory Center. Accessed December 07, 2020. http://www.thememorycenter.com/can-you-recover-from-alzheimers-or-dementia/.

"B.C. Alzheimer's patient will be fed despite statement of wishes." The Globe and Mail. March 25, 2019. Accessed December 08, 2017. https://www.theglobeandmail.com/news/british-columbia/court-rejects-argument-that-living-will-means-alzheimers-patient-shouldnt-be-fed/article23269433/.

"Fetal Pain: The Evidence." Doctors on Fetal Pain. N.p., n.d. Web. 28 July 2019. <http://www.doctorsonfetalpain.com/>.

3. Adverse Physical and Psychological Health Effects

How can neurological, visual, metabolic characteristics affect e-mental health? Physiological changes consisting of neurological, visual and metabolic alterations are all affected by the transition to conditions of increased exposure within the digital world. With the ever-so rapid advancements of technological innovations, society becomes more reliant on smart devices and artificial algorithms. Influences of technology in our modern world remain a multi-dimensional issue, and as such in the context of e-mental health, there exist multiple sides to be considered.

Adverse effects come hand-in-hand with the establishment of a tool that relies on technology. With an increase in screen-time, higher risk of leading to dependence and/or addictive behavior, and long-term problems that affect body metabolism and sleep, a long list of such effects accompany e-mental health despite its promise of betterment of emotional and psychological wellbeing. In fact, the move to a digital landscape has left us with the growing trend towards a sedentary lifestyle in contemporary society.

Perhaps the most common physiological change anticipated with the transition to e-mental health would be neurological modifications. Permanent changes in the brain have been previously observed with cases of technology overuse or dependence. Traditionally, addiction has been a pervasive concept in the context of drug abuse and gambling behavior. However, with the increase in 21st century gadgets and rapidly expansive growth of the internet, light is shed on addiction. Much of the neurophysiological changes to brain structure and function in the context of virtual addictions are quite similar to addiction with drug and opioid addictions. The white and grey matter of the brain shrink in size, thereby resulting in loss of interests, declines in emotional processing, and degradation of overall neural functions.

Dependence is second nature to any form of management. Perhaps various online addictions are the commonest causes of these disease states inherent to technology. The accompanying weight gain and loss, effects on sleep, and eye health are exemplified in common stereotypes in society. A variety of physiological symptoms can be elicited as signs of dependence. For example, carpal tunnel syndrome can result from excess typing, use of controls, or pressing of buttons in video games. Irritations to the eye, blurry vision, eye strain, headaches, and migraines can ensue prolonged periods of screentime. Negative effects can also follow as a consequence of sedentary lifestyle and habits. Mental health symptoms are perhaps more predominant and of larger concern for the overall well-being of individuals. For some, feelings of isolation are a common consequence of excessive use of virtual devices. For others, the loss of time and realization of wasted time brings about negative feelings of guilt and stress. When considering stresses, perhaps the largest category of mental health disorders associated with dependence is depression.

What we may often neglect as onlookers concerned by mental health are the expansive influences that transitioning to online delivery of services can have on physical health. We have seen examples of this in light of COVID-19, which predominated 2020. The rates of depression across the globe soared to a peak within this year. It may have been fear but it also may have been our transition to the virtual world for connections and seeking a place of belonging. For many, the activities they engage in the virtual world may be a solace or place to de-stress from an already stressful lifestyle. Despite this however, the isolation and loneliness brought about by extended periods of time in this digital reality could have more adverse effects to our mental health.

We might be able to paint a picture of this grim reality if we consider a psychodynamic perspective. We must not neglect grief and loss that individuals can face in a situation, where there is a complete lack of in-person interactions. Perhaps in his work on mourning and melancholia, Sigmund Freud captures the extent of depressive effects that technology by examining the divided psychosomatic response to loss by drawing a fine line between mourning, a conscious response characterized by grief, and melancholia, a form of pathological depression – where he provides a theoretical clinical report on the two types of emotions based on his observations. Freud implements a diagnostic approach characterizing both responses as a condition induced by the stimulus, loss. In our case, the loss can be a number of aspects - loss of connections, loss of one's sense of reality, loss of health, loss of happiness, etc.

In his analysis of these two states of mind, he radicalizes each to opposite extremities. He asserts mourning a wholly healthy response, the mind's natural inclination. On the other hand, he declares melancholia an adamant disease with symptoms that gradually consume self-esteem, depreciate individual worth and give rise to contemplations of suicide. Perhaps the most illustrative example of this in history can be observed in the Blue Whale Challenge phenomenon, which began in 2016. In what was said to be a 'social network game', users participated in a challenge where a series of tasks were assigned to players to complete over 50 days. First, the challenges were harmless. As the days progressed however, more and more tasks instructing self-harm and the production of proof associated with this was required. Finally, on the last day of the challenge, players were required to commit suicide. Over the years, several countries around the world connected suicides of children and young adults thought to be associated with games like the Blue Whale Challenge and similar ones. While not so explicit, incidents like this present the fragility of the human mind and intentional dangers of virtual world - though oftentimes, there are unintentional dangers as well.

Throughout his paper, Freud implies a message that individuals should recognize and adapt to accommodate loss rather than perpetually lamenting in a cycle of stasis; he postulates and portrays melancholia as a morbid delirium. Nonetheless, we must acknowledge he had claimed, "from the outset [to] drop all claim to general validity for our conclusions" as he most, if not all of his assertions, were mere speculations and unconfirmed truth. Nevertheless, though recognized as limited and flawed to a great extent, psychodynamic theory can help us to guide our understandings on these psychological effects of grief on the human mind. Freud develops conjectures in mourning, for instance, one remembers the loss which is "hyper-cathected, and detachment of libido is accomplished" yet "[t]he fact is…when the work of mourning is completed the ego becomes free and uninhibited again." (244) We can acknowledge effects of mourning are temporary and but melancholia can have a large effect on one's cathexis, libido and ego – all inherent to the Freudian psyche (McLeod 2013), which is a model constructed to embody such abstract theories that encompass Freud's subjective views. The intangible classifications of id, which is established as instinctual drives limited moderately by ego, and completely by superego, and libido as a form of energy deriving from id, displays his attempts to perhaps embody philosophical impressions and science concurrently. He makes statements regarding mourning and melancholia such as, "we found that the inhibition and loss of interest are fully accounted for by …mourning …[where] ego is absorbed" though there was neither experimentation nor observations to make such a finding.

In addition, his definition of the ego as an ambiguous, moderating entity enables him to comment on its imagined, symptom-absorbing propensities.

However, the conceptualization he offers his exhibition of philosophy as pseudo-psychology, present only the establishment of a stage to make ostensibly valid accusations against melancholia to strengthen perhaps a convoluted message. Despite this, Freud's portrayal disapproving prolonged stasis in response to a loss may very well capture extreme effects of dependence and loss of interactions in e-mental health. Melancholia is transformed from simply prolonged depression to "a hallucinatory wishful psychosis", (244) "self-tormenting…sadistic satisfaction", "psychogenic…mania", and a "cannibalistic phase", showing symptoms such as the "delusional expectation of punishment", "hysteria" and "schizophrenia". (248) Images of the ravaged, deteriorated mind provoke connotations of paranoia and hallucination, which though exaggerated, may give us a glimpse into the minds of individuals who are dependent in the digital world. When Freud refers to the attributes of melancholia, he alleges its connection to "phenomen[a] in obsessional neurosis", suggesting a clinical condition of sorts with a great link to depression and loss, which may have precisely been Freud's intent. His criticism of melancholia as "circular insanity" leading to a "circuitous path of self-punishment" (251) serves to refine his notions regarding lament, particularly the notion that prolonged melancholy from loss will only result in a state of immobility, in an emotional sense. He conveys that it is critical to move forward accepting the loss and persisting to live instead of contemplating on the loss. At its surface,

Freud's exposition is a presentation of his psycho-analytical theory but in reality, it conceals ideas regarding the futility of lamentation and the need to advance when one encounters a loss. Furthermore, while melancholia is certainly a pathological condition, Freud's division of melancholy and mourning based solely on a "certain lapse of time" (244) and strict segregation of these categories, carries the implication that remaining in stasis will only exhaust one's "libidinal investments", or plainly mental energy, and the best alternative is to reflect, and to progress. This gives us a space to deconstruct as we must understand the digital world can still be a healthy part of our lives, given that we act in moderation.

Both adverse physiological and mental health effects can characterize dependence in the digital world. These symptoms, though many are recognizable, may or may not present itself thereby making it difficult to discern within our society. COVID-19, instances of cyberbullying and abuse, and psychodynamic analysis of our states of mind have given us insights into how these adverse effects may manifest psychologically. Nevertheless, a healthy balance may be achievable.

References:
Freud, Sigmund. "Mourning and Melancholia." The Standard Edition of the Complete Psychological Works of Sigmund Freud 14 (1920): 243-58.English.upenn.edu. Hogarth Press, 2014. Web. 26 Feb. 2015.

Faigley, Lester, Roger Graves, and Heather Graves. The Brief Penguin Handbook, Third Canadian Edition. 3rd ed. Boston, MA: Pearson Custom Pub., 2013. Print.

McLeod, Saul. "Sigmund Freud's Theories - The Psyche." Simply Psychology. Simply Psychology, 2013. Web. 29 Feb. 2015. <http://www.simplypsychology.org/Sigmund-Freud.html>.

4. Cyberwars and e-mental health: what can we learn from the past?

Most of the conflict that has emerged in the history of human civilization is a result of the walls people create between themselves and when differences in ideology, beliefs, appearances, practices, customs, or some other aspect exist. Evgeny Morozov's statement, "[i]nformation technology has been one of the leading drivers of globalization, and it may also become one of its major victims," reflects the current state of affairs when we consider the conflict that exists online. What we have, presently, is a tool that enables us to open up barriers, which were once not there. Our mentalities are easily influenced and principles of inequality need to be considered in the context of e-mental health within our contemporary society. While it is true that we are able to bring the world together through globalization, and thus have the capacity for greater accessibility, it is nevertheless the fact of the matter that there exist problems that can aggravate or lead to further conflicts.

The divergence created by the digital divide gives us a glimpse into the between-individuals disparities that spark conflict within and between societies. Historically, we have observed gatekeeping, which offers us an example of the conflicts that disparities in access to information can create. Namely, we see that powerful individuals would control propaganda and filter what information gets to which group of people.

Perhaps the underlying principle is more evident in nature: speciation forms distinct biological species over time because of geographical, behavioral, physiological or other biological barriers. In an analogous case in Central America several centuries ago, a species of shrimps were isolated by geographical barriers and after having diverged into separate species were placed together. These two species had, as members of the same species, once courted peacefully. After becoming two discrete species however, they demonstrated violent aggression towards one other when reintroduced into the same environment. The same can be applied to human aggression and conflict as similar principles extend, by way of nature.

If the conception of this barrier were extended to the digital divide, the seclusion of two sets of subjects regardless of population size would cause each group to undergo subtle or immense change due to any range of variables. Let us consider the most obvious, which is the divide seen between that of the developing and developed world. For over 50 years, the developed world has faced a technological gap, while the developed world has evolved to the extent that innovations become obsolete in one or two years. In addition to novel communication styles, understandings, ideologies about the world, and value systems, people of the developing world will experience a culture shock were this barrier to be suddenly lifted after a significant duration of division. Not only would the interactions between the developed and developing world bring about a clash in values and perspectives, we should also be concerned about its impact on their beliefs, values, culture, and mental health being exposed to this new stream of information. There has already been iniquitousness in the allocation of resources, but now we provide an environment that risks a higher prospect for conflict than in their initial interaction.

Protracting this analogy, we must recognize that breaking the walls of the digital divide have both benefits and detriments. Globalization can provide access to services that better one's mental health regardless of the divide. Services once only offered in a certain location can now be accessed by others elsewhere. Likewise, one can now expand businesses, educate oneself and gain extensive knowledge, connect or build relationships with distant friends or family, and become closer as global citizens. Nevertheless, this closeness may open the door for conflicts, division, and its consequences that very often tend to originate from inadvertence, contrary views, malice, greed, extremism and other factors – all of which are present in the online environment. Thus, the offering of services and e-mental health of global citizens mandate that globalization is taken into account.

Unintentional harm and miscommunication, two concepts perhaps inherent to conceptual innovations that can have a massive influence on e-mental health, and thereby easily transform into an incessant cycle of retribution. Take for instance the time when the United States (US) placed an oil embargo on Japan during the Second World War, a declaration of war was delivered in Japanese. Without an adequate intermediary and due to the language barrier, it was interpreted to be their notice of withdrawal from the war and request for the lifting of oil embargos. Thus, the Japanese attack on Pearl Harbor in 1941 was regarded unwarranted and swept a wave of outrage among American citizens. Conflict heightened significantly as the US retaliated violently against their opposing forces in World War II. The US's response attack on Pearl Harbor was not only a result of miscommunication but also due to American nationalism and affiliation in the Allied Forces, a military alliance during the war against the Axis powers, which Japan was a member of. The conflict was due to not only the geographical barriers between them but also the psychological walls created from their allegiance solely to their nation and alliance. This division enabled both nations to commit these atrocities resulting in crippling casualties for both sides. The wall blinded both groups and catalyzed the result leading to the "major victims" that described by Morozov.

Now let's consider this same scenario in the digital world, where a constant stream of information continues to bombard us, where we are not aware of which sources to trust or how to translate the language within different environments online. What are the effects on mental health consequent to us lifting the walls and barriers, enabling miscommunication? Despite measures to protect anonymity and privacy, we have seen time and time again that such notions may very well be non-existent. In fact, we must recognize that the digital divide, globalization, and privacy concerns only touch the surface of the kind of implications associated with and intrinsic to novel technologies.

Over the course of time, separate groups become divided by distinct ideologies, cultural values and beliefs, or even human greed and maliciousness which stem from geographical, ideological, and various forms of inequality – perhaps the epitome of what we see on many online servers today. Consider the 2020 cyberattacks on the US government by Russian hackers. By sneaking a malicious code onto Orion, a popular software, hackers breached into the system to steal information from the energy, commerce, treasury and state sectors, ultimately threatening state cyber security. Regardless of the intent, it is possible for such conflicts to arise digitally much like the physical world. The consequences in this setting may lead to the loss of privacy, information security, and the demise of nations - though in a different way than in wars. Perhaps one such occasion in history, where a parallel can be observed, was when views collided during the period of the Cold War between 1945 and 1991. The US headed the Western world and the Soviet Union dominated the Eastern world. Since both nations possessed nuclear weapons capable of a nuclear holocaust, most of the conflicts between the nations were proxy wars within other regions between groups indoctrinated with the Soviet Union's ideology of socialism and collectives following the liberal democracy ideology of the US. One significant event was the establishment of the Berlin Wall drawing a line between East and West Berlin. The creation of this border demonstrates the Soviet Union's desire to reaffirm walls that existed before the conflict. The elimination of the geographical and psychological barrier resulted in an ideological war. The overlapping of political dogmas led the conflict, the means to proclaim one correct ideology. These proxy wars can, without a doubt, extend to technological spheres as well. How then would this look like?

One example may be the loss, theft, fraud, and legal concerns we have seen with the emergence of cryptocurrency. With the rise of bitcoin and other cryptocurrencies, the ability for criminals to exploit anonymity and enable laundering of money through the web has become clear. Perhaps a paramount driver for a cyberwar is the human greed for power and/or a desire to create some form of equality; this is a belief consistent in history. Before advances in technology, imperialism from the late nineteenth century to early twentieth century had influenced several nations within the world. The conquests for the expansion of colonies and power led German and Belgian imperialism to plant the seeds for conflicts within the nation of Rwanda. Legacies of the implemented hierarchies ignited the genocide of billions of Tutsis in what came to be known as the Rwandan genocide. The psychological barrier that was created in the case of cryptocurrencies and anonymity provided to individuals are similar to that created by the imperialists of Germany and Belgium. Generally, anonymity on servers are meant to protect privacy; at the same time however, this power enables the creation of hierarchies and systematic division which can lead to conflict and huge losses. Perhaps technology works to help remove some barriers but we must recognize that certain barriers hide inherent differences among people, which may ultimately lead to unwanted psychological consequences when they are exposed.

Though conditional, perhaps a theme we can learn from history and apply to the digital world is that conflict arises from the differences a dividing wall creates over time and then the sudden lifting of barriers or exposure to novel ideologies. The protection of mental health online therefore depends on both, the elimination of these barriers that are creating virtual apartheids in a slow, gradual, and careful manner. It also depends on the redefinition of what the walls are in e-mental health, telemedicine, and online. Perhaps the solution lies in the creation of permanent cooperative networks that all members of the world can be part of and at the same time reach an agreement on. Today, the United Nations offers the closest modern model to this network and the accommodation of many voices in the physical world. Perhaps we need a system of governance in the online world as well. Although some solutions require the establishment of certain barriers online to prevent conflict, we may need these barriers to be semi-permeable to the flow of information based on ethical principles and standards that are consistent with shared beliefs about universal care. As we have observed time and time again in history, global acceptance and principles of accommodation are vital for the development of a world without conflict online.

5. E-mental Health Tool: Clinical VR

The Role of Clinical VR

Virtual reality (VR) and augmented reality have drastically changed the way we view therapies for mental health disorders and rehabilitation. As VR engineers strive to produce more immersive experiences for users, it provides an appealing distraction, permitting people to "lose" themselves in the world of VR. People are so engaged that they do not notice what's happening peripherally in their surroundings and may lose track of the time that has passed. One application that this immersion can largely benefit is in the context of monitoring patients in rehabilitation environments (Whalley, 1995). In this setting, patients will be able to experience and pursue pleasures while researchers and clinicians obtain the relevant data they need.

For example, quite recently, a tech company called VRHealth launched their new artificial intelligence (AI) trainer called Luna – a cognitive behaviour therapy (CBT) program for pain management in seniors("VRHealth, AARP launch VR platform for remote patient monitoring, in-home therapy | MobiHealthNews," n.d.). Through its VR-directed programming, Luna will be able to "help seniors receive therapist-guided physical therapy without needing to leave their home." While, theoretically, this sounds like an exceptional idea – this scenario is fraught with problems. Throughout this chapter, we will be considering some of the ulterior motives and issues that ought to be considered alongside this exciting development. Before entering this discussion, there ought to be a disclaimer that this will be a large degree of speculation involved.

Conflicts of Interest

1. Researcher agendas

Firstly, there is a likelihood that there is a conflict of interest for researchers. As those who develop VR and knowledge leaders in this area become eager to push such technologies forward, several ethical concerns come into play. Firstly, the researcher may push their own agendas to further research while disregarding patient autonomy. For example, a huge part of CBT and other exposure therapies are that these strategies are reliant on the patient confronting specific alterations that are introduced as stimuli. Perhaps this is best illustrated by work done in VR exposure therapy for patients with post-traumatic stress disorder (PTSD)(Kothgassner et al., 2019). The problem with PTSD along with phobias and addictions are that the participants or patients of the VR program are subjected to mentally perceived harmful stimuli. As such, it can serve to worsen symptoms of their phobias and addictions, should they be re-exposed to it with enough realism. Furthermore, the concept of informed consent becomes blurred. As researchers may chose to take decisions for them, the patients or participants are prevented from opportunities to provide informed consent and withdrawal from participation.

2.   Corporate agendas

Similarly, with independent companies commercializing VR technology for remote rehabilitation, a new level of partnership must be reached as hospitals, clinics, and educational institutions rely on corporate support. This may mean that certain services and products will only be provided if medical professionals promote them to patients.

Another area of potential concern arises from data companies that control or store patient data. As these corporate entities act as the intermediaries for perhaps highly confidential patient data, are there proper laws and security systems in place to control them? For example, consider the Focus on Therapeutic Outcomes Inc. (FOTO) corporation. It is a hugely successful and widely implemented outcomes management system used for measuring functional orthopedic patient outcome measures. With a patient base over 26 million, the company supports roughly 25,000 clinicians. Many companies, just like FOTO, have been able to show the growing potential that can be tapped into in terms of the remote patient performance monitoring software market.

Although most of these companies use wearable devices, this represents a likely pathway for VR object deployment as well. This means that VR therapies and interventions could eventually become commercial and like in many privatized healthcare models, it could become a treatment option only accessible for the elite few.

However, regardless of the integrity of these corporate entities, the concern remains about cybersecurity of health data. For instance, there was an unsuccessful recent cyberattack against the United States Department of Health and Human Services. To provide a bit more context, the United States has a system that relies heavily on having electronic records for health as a result of the rules and regulations outlined by the Centres of Medicare and Medicaid Services. This is because of the Health Insurance Portability and Accountability Act legislation. This underlines the importance of needing more robust systems to support the safety and confidentiality of patient data within the healthcare system.

3.   Lack of Supervisory decision-making

Secondly, a lack of human feedback can be harmful, especially when considering the previous example of CBT. The fact that clinicians are hampered from interfering with a program that is largely machine-driven can mean that the clinicians would not be able to step in and withdraw the intervention provided there're cues that indicate they cannot participate. While it can be argued that the AI can make this decision for them using cues within the system – it may be hard for the patient or family caregiver at home to perceive when it is necessary to disengage from VR.

Similarly, during this research period, the AI is trained with a plethora of stimuli that will be provided by sample patients. If there are rare, specific patient-centred needs that arise, it would take a longer period of time to train. We cannot ignore that there is a risk that patients may be given directives that actually lead to more harm than benefit.

Replacing healthcare jobs

The idea that you can have a virtual physical therapist that can supersede human ones inherently leads to the question: why do we even need human physical therapists in the first place? This is a bold statement and perhaps it will take years or decades to reach this level, but it still ought to be thought about. In this case, perhaps inevitably it'll lead to a decrease in specialized professions like this one as knowledge becomes offloaded onto servers and the cloud. With the loss of such specialties, perhaps novel types of professions will also effervesce forth. As these types of programs are being developed, more engineers and technical skill-oriented professions will be needed to support the complex demands of the patient.

Loss of social presence

With the lack of physical therapists, there is a likelihood that patients are not given the same level of encouragement or human elements of interaction. For example, face-to-face communication would be replaced with avatars and audio prompts in headsets. Regardless of how realistic the VR may be, the patient is denied the ability to socialize and receive more sensitive counsel from a human physical therapist.

Additionally, the immersion can lead to feelings of embodiment in VR that can further socially isolate patients. As graphic designers become better at reducing uncanny valley effects in VR, these may be accompanied by a distortion of reality. Patients may come to depend excessively on the VR program and not want to do these activities in their functional world. After all, performing activities and monitoring them in VR quantitatively is limited to the number of sensors that can be fitted on the patient. Self-reports and other subjective measures can be biased without the presence of a white coat figure.

The trend seemingly approaches closer to a world where virtual clinics are the norm, especially in light of recent events. As more people become wary of infection and spread of disease, virtual clinics are truly advantageous in that they can prevent the incidence of more diseases while offering patients care, albeit a less effective means of it, via digital interfaces. However, what role can VR play in offering this type of care?
This is where other forms of VR can play a role, such as augmented reality (AR). AR is a form of holographic projection that has been renowned in the field of surgery for allowing surgeons and other specialists to visualize skeletons or anatomical landmarks for treatment.

Technological Gap

As VR can be considered to still be in its infancy, there are several regions across the globe that are under-resourced and can be systemically excluded from partaking in the same opportunities bestowed by VR. Resultantly, there has been an attempt to use low-cost VR that has been greatly bolstered by the advancements made in PC hardware over the last decade. Higher graphics processing power and VR hardware such as untethered Oculus head-mounted displays have significantly revolutionized the ability of the everyday user to purchase reasonably priced hardware for VR. The availability of powerful PC engines and 3D accelerator graphics cards allow

VR PCs to process and display
in 3D in real-time.

There is not doubt that immersion is becoming more affordable. Collectively, these advancements of computing power efficiency have provided for developers to create more compelling simulations in price ranges under $1000. In hindsight, the cost of head mounted displays a decade ago was 10-20 times more costly. If trends continue, chances are that these prices are likely to decline even further in the next few years. VR software has also greatly improved over the last decade with the ability to manipulate 3D objects and mimic visual, audio and even haptic feedback. Some software toolkits are even available for free (Alice WTK). With code and software development kits becoming increasingly open access, the capabilities of the average programmer are significantly increased. With this, issues around intellectual property, plagiarism, and database management persist.

Another innovation that has allowed for low-cost VR to be useful is the development of VR Modeling Language. The VRML is a growingly widespread programming language that is a 3D graphics file format and run-time description for use on the World Wide Web, including interactive and animated elements that can be interfaced with Java and JavaScript scripting languages, both of which are commonly employed by web programmers.

Applications of low-cost VR and VRML for telemedicine are becoming increasingly apparent. Particularly, VR can be used for interactive visualization of 3D fields and inexpensive workstations using VRML. This allows clinicians to interactively engage with a patient that could be geographically distant from hub locations. It could even be used to completely remove the clinician from the equation. Instead, the created VR objects may choose to have virtual "clinicians" that relay instructions and feedback for a treatment plan.(Riva & Gamberini, 2000)

However, how would an error with the VR technology be dealt with? Faulty graphics, an error in detection, or other ineffective technical glitches, as infrequent as they may be, ought to be addressed. This is the reason why the question of technical support and having clinicians either a) work alongside engineers or b) be equipped with specialized training to support technical concerns is essential.

Health Effects

As VR objects are introduced into the lives of those in the clinical setting (patients, healthcare practitioner, support staff), the safety and ethical issues of VR are introduced as well. Some well-documented concerns of the side effects of prolonged exposures (dependent on the persons' susceptibility) to VR environments are:

- Motion sickness;

- Ocular system strain;

- Degraded postural and limb control;

- Reduced sense of presence;

- Negative compensatory responses that can train injurious or extraneous compensatory responses.

That being said, curbing these health effects are one of the goals of VR engineers and developers. Over the course of the last decade, these side effects have been effectively reduced and made actual reports of simulation sickness next to negligible. However, this is in no way underplaying the risk because the demographic of patients that are being exposed to such treatment may be particularly vulnerable.

For instance, one popular application of VR is its use in CBT. Recently, there have been studies such as the clinical trials being done in military veterans diagnosed with post-traumatic stress disorder (PTSD) on clinical exposure to a stress-inducing stimulus as a part of exposure therapy. (Van Den Berg et al., 2015) In situations like this, it becomes of utmost importance that the graphics and visual renditioning of said stimuli are portrayed realistically.

Noting that the way that CBT typically works is by exposing the patient to progressively stronger presentations of the stimulus until they are desensitized to elicit the fear response, there are multiple possible risks associated with the VR simulation. In the less serious instance, we can consider a possibly less serious version of the stress-inducing stimulus. For illustrative purposes, suppose it is the sound of a gunshot firing at a faraway distance. If the patient is consistently exposed to lower intensities of such a stimulus, chances are that the patient's shell shock may not be effectively curbed, but it does not lead to unwarranted harm or injury to the patient. However, consider if the patient is exposed to something more serious a bit too early in the treatment. For example, the graphic designer of the VR object may have added some graphic effects that were a bit too exaggerated and coupled perfectly with a grenade explosion at close quarters. This can lead to the patient being traumatized and non-compliant to continue future interventions or even lead to more drastic PTSD symptoms. Although this example is hyperbolic, it remains that it is difficult for scientists and engineers to determine exactly where to draw the line.

The implementation of VR in remote patient monitoring is an exciting development and one that should be carefully thought about prior to widespread adoption. This chapter draws attention to some of the drawbacks that can arise as a result.

References
Kothgassner, O. D., Goreis, A., Kafka, J. X., Van Eickels, R.

L., Plener, P. L., & Felnhofer, A. (2019). Virtual reality exposure therapy for posttraumatic stress disorder (PTSD): a meta-analysis. European Journal of Psychotraumatology, Vol. 10. https://doi.org/10.1080/20008198.2019.1654782

Riva, G., & Gamberini, L. (2000). Virtual reality in telemedicine. Telemedicine Journal, 6(3), 327–340. https://doi.org/10.1089/1530562200750040183

Van Den Berg, D. P. G., De Bont, P. A. J. M., Van Der Vleugel, B. M., De Roos, C., De Jongh, A., Van Minnen, A., & Van Der Gaag, M. (2015). Prolonged exposure vs eyemovement desensitization and reprocessing vs waiting list for posttraumatic stress disorder in patients with a psychotic disorder: A randomized clinical trial. JAMA Psychiatry, 72(3), 259–267. https://doi.org/10.1001/jamapsychiatry.2014.2637

VRHealth, AARP launch VR platform for remote patient monitoring, in-home therapy | MobiHealthNews. (n.d.). Retrieved March 28, 2020, from https://www.mobihealthnews.com/content/vrhealth-aarp-launch-vr-platform-remote-patient-monitoring-home-therapy

Whalley, L. J. (1995). Ethical issues in the application of virtual reality to medicine. Computers in Biology and Medicine, 25(2), 107–114. https://doi.org/10.1016/0010-4825(95)00008-R

6: The Future of Mental Health in the Era of COVID-19

The SARS-CoV-2 pandemic has led to worldwide stay-at-home orders and social isolation. Despite the lack of research exploring the potential influence of loneliness and isolation on the severity of SARS-CoV-2, studies have related loneliness and isolation to factors directly attributing to aggravating the severity of SARS-CoV-2. Although there are many factors that contribute to severe illness from SARS-CoV-2, taking measures to reduce the feeling of isolation may serve as a viable prevention measure.

COVID-19 and Mental Health

COVID-19 and quarantine measures have posed an unprecedented burden on mental health of Canadians, across all demographics. With the new demands of remote operation, everyone from parents to policymakers to pandemic workers in the front-line are left susceptible to spikes in their level of anxiety and stress.

Decreased social supports during self-isolation among other factors can be attributable for the rise in addictions. The overall emotional states during quarantine of confusion, frustration, and boredom push people to escapist outlets that may quickly turn to dependency.

With children and other dependents stuck at home, quarantine prevents them from social engagement, experiential learning, and positive psychosocial interactions to take place. This negatively affects their growth and can result in societal retrogradation.

Many studies have also reported post-traumatic stress disorder symptoms as a putative challenge in isolation. Stressors such as quarantine duration, infection paranoia, and lack of resources can induce long-lasting effects on a person's psyche.

COVID-19 and Loneliness

Despite the lack of research exploring the potential influence of loneliness and isolation on the severity of SARS-CoV-2, studies have shown that loneliness and isolation contribute to factors directly attributing to aggravating the severity of SARS-CoV-2 (Minotti et al., 2020; Novotney Amy, 2019;CDC, 2020; Zheng et al., 2020) . These studies have demonstrated an association between isolation, lowered immune response, higher inflammation markers, cardiovascular disease, and risk for diabetes (Minotti et al., 2020; CDC, 2020; Zheng et al., 2020). Although there are many factors that contribute to severe illness from SARS-CoV-2, taking measures to reduce the feeling of isolation may serve as a viable prevention measure.

The innate immune system is significant in preparing the body for adaptive immunity and swiftly killing virally infected cells and preparing a more specific immune response through adaptive immunity such as antibodies. Several studies focused on the innate immunity of isolated groups, lonely groups versus non-isolated, and non-lonely groups have seen deleterious effects on the immunity of lonely and isolated groups.

A study of elderly rats that were isolated for 8 weeks found a significantly lower natural killer (NK) cell activity and proliferation response of lymphocytes (Cruces et al., 2014). A similar finding of a decline in NK cell activity was reported by studies in lonely medical students and psychiatric inpatients (Kiecolt-Glaser, Garner, et al., 1984; Kiecolt-Glaser, Ricker, et al., 1984). NK cells are known to kill virally infected cells as part of the innate immune response and release antiviral cytokines such as IFN-γ (Eissmann Philipp, n.d.). In fact, deficiencies in NK cells have been associated with increased viral susceptibility (Eissmann Philipp, n.d.). Hence, a lack of these cells prior to a viral infection such as SARS-CoV-2 would not be ideal as the immune system would need to rely on other immune mechanisms to fight the infection.

However, some literature has suggested that immunocompromised individuals are not as prone to a severe course of infection (Minotti et al., 2020), thus this point still needs to be further researched. Nonetheless, several studies have found a positive association between loneliness, weaker immune system, and severe SARS-CoV-2 prognosis. Furthermore, DNA microarray analysis has shown downregulation of regulatory genes supporting type I interferon responses and mature B lymphocyte function (Cole et al., 2007) in lonelier individuals. Type I interferons and B lymphocytes from part of the innate immune response. Analysis of NK cell function using peripheral blood samples from SARS-CoV-2 patients found an inverse correlation between disease severity and NK cell levels (Zheng et al., 2020).

As noted earlier, increased severity of SARS-CoV-2 is associated with increased inflammatory cytokines. In this area, there have also been a series of studies in both animal models and humans that show a link in increased inflammatory cytokines, and loneliness and isolation. Compared to those feeling more socially connected, lonelier people have been reported to have increased MCP-1 (Hackett et al., 2012), up-regulation of pro-inflammatory genes, increased cytokines including IL-6, and TNF-α (Jaremka et al., 2013). Even so, psychological stressors have also been associated with higher counts of TNF-α and IL-6 (Jaremka et al., 2013). While the presented studies are not directly linked to the inflammation seen in severe cases of SARS-CoV-2, these studies show an increase in the same inflammatory cytokines related to severe illness from SARS-CoV-2. Similarly, high levels of these same cytokines have been related to other diseases. In all these studies, there were significantly lower levels of inflammatory cytokines in the non-lonely, and non-isolated groups

E-Mental Health Access
Unfortunately, there is still an unbridged gap between

the supply and demand of mental health resources both short-term and long-term. This is where E-mental health service delivery can shine.

If physicians, social workers, and other healthcare professionals can make the transition to start offering counseling and other mental health services remotely via mobile apps and the web, it will significantly reduce transport times and person-to-person infection rates.

However, even long-standing service providers are facing challenges. For example, Kids Help Phone has served as the national helpline for youths for over 30 years. However, the onset of the pandemic has swamped the distress service with calls and texts from adults as well. Ironically, reduced bandwidth places service staff at a higher risk of youth contracting mental illness.

Online self-help platforms and forums are providing those struggling with depression and anxiety the opportunity to connect with like-minded people and support each other. This represents a way to lower the burden on healthcare professionals particularly in relation to those struggling from the "quarantine blues" (as opposed to those with more serious mental health conditions).

Technology has also changed the way mental health services can be accessed, which is especially important during COVID-19. For example, there are several mobile mental health services that operate through text messages – a simple but effective concept. There are more sophisticated apps that also collect information on a user's typical behaviour and provide a signal when there is a change in this behaviour. There are services available to connect individuals to peer counsellors or health care professionals. Specifically, telepsychotherapy is the best known form of E-mental health. The power of digital technologies must be harnessed to improve access to and effectiveness of treatment. During COVID-19, the feelings of anxiety and loneliness have increased the need for mental health services. Thus, teleconsultations have become the new normal (Vial, 2020).

However, prior to the pandemic, there was already a lack of tele-mental health solutions that could be used for psychiatrists, but a surge in non-scientifically based mental health apps. The success of these apps is not necessarily tied to the pandemic, but results from the growing demand for this type of healthcare. Headspace and Insight Timer have been some of the most commonly used wellness apps during this time. They provide free guided meditations that have introduced people of all ages to some strategies that promote mental well-being (NIMH, 2020). In addition, there are several online anxiety and depression support groups online, such as Turn2Me, which hosts free sessions run by qualified professionals. This network has also offered sessions to help people specifically cope with the dread of COVD-19 (Kindelan, 2020).

It's evident that COVID-19 came as a shock to most of the population. An event that causes such a drastic change in our way of life is bound to have psychological impacts. The lockdowns that have been initialized worldwide undoubtedly resulted in people having intense feelings of loneliness, anxiety, and a general altered worldview. This led many people to turn to technology as an escape and a coping mechanism. The use of technology in the form of online shopping and several social media platforms has the ability to cause heightened feelings of depression and loneliness. On the other hand, platforms such as TikTok have been utilized to spread positive messages, and the increase in mental health resources online has allowed individuals to adequately cope with the current situation. In times of distress and confusion, this pandemic has shown us that we must have faith in our global community to find solutions to the problems we face, from the physical spread of the virus to the psychological problems associated with social distancing.

Education on Providing Clinical Care Virtually

It is equally important that the quality of mental health care is not compromised. This is where proper psychoeducation becomes crucial. It is important people offer help with tact and sensitivity, however there are limited figurative and sometimes literal bandwidths for using tech.

Alberta Health Services is leading a campaign of mental health initiatives in response to COVID-19, alongside its work to digitize health records via Connect Care. Extensive education efforts are being made by healthcare professionals to master the user interfaces of these mobile and digital tools.

Confidentiality and Anonymity Online

Mental health concerns, by nature, tend to be intensely private. Body image issues, drinking problems, sexuality – some of the most personal topics can be veiled by online anonymity. No one necessarily needs to know one's identity prior to offering adequate care.

However, this also comes with limitations, as anonymity breeds mischief. Can health users of such services be exposed to illegitimate sources of fraud? Yes. Can legitimate health platforms be met with users that abuse the system? Yes. Fortunately, there are unique digital identifiers that can be used to curb these problems. That being said, these identifiers become loaded with a person's medical information and can become a source of concern. With cyberattacks and insecure databases, there exists concerns of online data storage sites being hacked. This warrants healthcare systems to try to find and purchase systems to protect the data at a time when the sector is already facing significant resource challenges.

A Positive Note

The good news is that if these tools are properly used, there are ways to reduce the biggest complaint of our healthcare system: time and effort. Waiting and travel times often frustrate and even prevent people from seeking out help. If online and digital modes of healthcare delivery become the norm, perhaps the stigmas and hesitations to go see a psychiatrist, social worker, or other healthcare professional will reduce.

References
Cole, S. W., Hawkley, L. C., Arevalo, J. M., Sung, C. Y., Rose, R. M., & Cacioppo, J. T. (2007b). Social regulation

of gene expression in human leukocytes. Genome Biology, 8(9). https://doi.org/10.1186/gb-2007-8-9-r189

Cruces, J., Venero, C., Pereda-Pérez, I., & De la Fuente, M. (2014). A higher anxiety state in old rats after social isolation is associated to an impairment of the immune response. Journal of Neuroimmunology, 277(1–2), 18–25. https://doi.org/10.1016/j.jneuroim.2014.09.011

Eissmann Philipp. (n.d.). Natural Killer Cells | British Society for Immunology. Retrieved August 27, 2020, from https://www.immunology.org/public-information/bite-sizedimmunology/cells/natural-killer-cells

Hackett, R. A., Hamer, M., Endrighi, R., Brydon, L., & Steptoe, A. (2012). Loneliness and stress-related inflammatory and neuroendocrine responses in older men and women. Psychoneuroendocrinology, 37(11), 1801–1809. https://doi.org/10.1016/j.psyneuen.2012.03.016

Jaremka, L. M., Fagundes, C. P., Peng, J., Bennett, J. M., Glaser, R., Malarkey, W. B., & Kiecolt-Glaser, J. K. (2013). Loneliness Promotes Inflammation During Acute Stress. Psychological Science, 24(7), 1089–1097. https://doi.org/10.1177/0956797612464059

Kiecolt-Glaser, J. K., Garner, W., Speicher, C., Penn, G. M., Holliday, J., & Glaser, R. (1984). Psychosocial modifiers of immunocompetence in medical students. Psychosomatic Medicine, 46(1), 7–14. https://doi.org/10.1097/00006842-198401000-00003

Kiecolt-Glaser, J. K., Ricker, D., George, J., Messick, G., Speicher, C. E., Garner, W., & Glaser, R. (1984). Urinary cortisol levels, cellular immunocompetency, and loneliness in psychiatric inpatients. Psychosomatic Medicine, 46(1), 15–23. https://doi.org/10.1097/00006842-198401000-00004

Kindelan, K. (2020, April 6). 8 Apps to Support your Mental Health. Retrieved August 09, 2020, from https://abcnews.go.com/gma/wellness/apps-support-mental-health-mindfulness/story?id=55890971

Minotti, C., Tirelli, F., Barbieri, E., Giaquinto, C., & Donà, D. (2020a). How is immunosuppressive status affecting children and adults in SARS-CoV-2 infection? A systematic review. In Journal of Infection (Vol. 81, Issue 1, pp. e61–e66). W.B. Saunders Ltd. https://doi.org/10.1016/j.jinf.2020.04.026

NIMH. (2020). Technology and the Future of Mental Health Treatment. Retrieved August 09, 2020, from https://www.nimh.nih.gov/health/topics/technology-and-the-future-of-mental-health-treatment/index.shtml

Vial, S. (2020, June 19). Coronavirus: New technologies can help maintain mental health in times of crisis. Retrieved August 09, 2020, from https://theconversation.com/coronavirus-new-technologies-can-help-maintain-mental-health-in-times-of-crisis-136576

Zheng, M., Gao, Y., Wang, G., Song, G., Liu, S., Sun, D., Xu, Y., & Tian, Z. (2020). Functional exhaustion of antiviral lymphocytes in COVID-19 patients. In Cellular and Molecular Immunology (Vol. 17, Issue 5, pp. 533–535). Springer Nature.

7. Privacy and Confidentiality

Introduction
Integrating technology into mental health can have many positive outcomes for medical professionals and patients. E-mental health includes the many types of technology which can be used in diagnosing and treating mental health issues. While there are many benefits in terms of ability to reach clients and provide quick assistance, privacy and confidentiality concerns can be complicated and provide significant drawbacks for e-mental health. Before deciding whether to utilize e-mental health services, an understanding of the risks is important. Both patients and mental health professionals must understand the security and privacy issues which exist when mental health treatment is taken into an online space. Only by being educated on e-mental health privacy concerns, regulations and steps to mitigate risk can users feel confident sharing private details regarding their mental health concerns.

Benefits
E-mental health comes with several benefits. Some of these benefits include reaching patients who live far

from healthcare providers, and the ability to help people when they need assistance without having to wait for an appointment. Additionally, e-mental health can provide aid in a diverse set of languages to help reach people who may feel a language barrier makes traditional treatment difficult. E-mental health can also provide a cost-effective option for areas where mental health services are costly. While each benefit e-mental health services bring are incredibly positive for those requiring mental health services, there are privacy and security risks involved with integrating technology into mental health.

Ethical Concerns

As the number of e-mental health service providers has increased steadily, ethical concerns have been raised. According to the paper titled Psychologists' ethical responsibilities in Internet-based groups: Issues, strategies and a call for dialogue, one ethical concern is the lack of clear jurisdiction which is created when a patient looks to online resources for mental health assistance. Local face-to-face treatment may be a better option for tailored help within an individual patients community (Humphreys et. al, 2000). The second concern addressed, is the difficulty of identifying someone in an online environment, and the possibility of patients impersonating other people. While some e-mental health programs utilize screen names to encourage anonymity, some traditional mental health providers integrate e-mental health into their existing offices. When conversing with patients outside the office, ensuring the correct individual is the person being spoken to is incredibly important. Should someone impersonate someone else online to a mental health professional, confidential information may be shared with the wrong person without a doctor knowing. Lastly, privacy in online conversations cannot be guaranteed to the same degree traditional mental health treatment can. To combat these ethical issues, guidelines are available in several countries which outline methods to create a safe environment for e-mental health patients. For example, legislation or professional associations may dictate confidentiality requirements, software safety or provide information for providing e-mental health programs outside a traditional office space. Tips for creating a safe environment will also be discussed within this chapter, along with information for users of e-mental health services.

Federal Privacy Policy

Each country will have their own policies and laws in place to protect the privacy and personal information of citizens. In Canada, each province has their own legislation, but at a federal level The Privacy Act and The Personal Information Protection and Electronic Documents Act governs the access of personal information and how the information can be handled and collected (McGrath et al., 2018). The Privacy Act gives citizens the right to view and correct any personal information the Government of Canada has collected, or any institutions subject to the act. The Personal Information Protection and Electronic Documents Act (PIPEDA) applies to private sector organizations and sets out legislation to regulate how information is collected and shared. Any medical professional wanting to branch into e-mental health must consult applicable government regulation to ensure confidentiality and appropriate handling of data.

Medical Device Regulations

Medical devices must typically meet criteria created by the government to ensure the safety of users. Apps are considered a medical device and are likely subject to legislation and regulations when being used for e-mental health purposes to protect patients. The number of health-related apps has exploded in recent years. In 2017, over 300 000 apps aimed to improve health were available (McGrath et al., 2018), which creates a market which is difficult to regulate. Regulation boards must balance the need to protect the public, with the need to allow innovation to help those in need. In Canada, Health Canada's Medical Devices Bureau of the Therapeutic Products Directorate (TPD), is responsible for monitoring and evaluating medical devices, including health apps. Each medical device is classified into four classes based on potential risk, with Class I being the lowest potential risk level to Class IV which is the highest potential risk in a medical device in Canada. Each class is subject to regulations and licensing requirements in order to become available to Canadian patients. All medical devices must be reviewed and pass layers of regulations in order to be available in the Canadian health market, and this includes health apps being available to Canadian citizens.

Professional Associations

Another type of regulation in place in Canada involves professional associations and regulatory bodies. In Canada, individual industries and individual provinces have regulatory associations which people who want to work within the industry, must become a member of and pass specific requirements. Within these existing organizations, like the Canadian Counselling and Psychotherapy Association, guidelines for the professional handling of patient data is typically included in the standards members must uphold. As e-health opportunities are increasing, electronic data handling and confidentiality is being included within the professional associations and their individual policies and standards. Those who work with e-mental health technologies are subject to the same legal standards as if the information were obtained in a traditional setting, and professional associations can help enforce the standards of professionalism in their accredited members.

Organizational Policies

While government regulation and professional associations can create a specific framework for handling sensitive information, each individual organization will decide on policies for their individual employees within the existing legal framework. When creating organizational policies, there are many areas which can be included for e-mental health use. One area which may be considered the most important, is to include all regulations and applicable laws for the country or area where the organization will be practicing. By branching out into an online space, new legislation may be applicable and needs to be communicated to staff working in e-mental health. Another area which should be included in an organizations policy regarding e-mental health is an overview of what information needs to be kept confidential. While this outline may exist for mental health treatment facilities already, when adding an online component, staff may need additional information regarding confidentiality. In addition to keeping client information private, an organization may want to include password privacy in their organizational policies. When an organization enters an e-mental health space, policies may want to be updated to include details regarding password strength and the frequency of changing passwords. Storing data electronically may be a concern for an organization. Data must be backed up, or saved in a second location, in the event of system error. While a backup may include a physical memory drive which would need to back up manually at specific intervals, it is much more likely that the software being used will have backups in place which are held online and do not require manual backup. Checking if files and information are adequately backed up is an important step and may need to be included in an organizations policy. Additionally, the safety of the backed-up material will be important to confirm. If backing up information seems complex, an information technologist can assist. If clients are contacting mental health assistance through social media, emailing or texting, staff will need to have some guidelines regarding the use of each method, and which employees would have access to which communication channel. Limiting access to those who need to have access is another step an organization can choose to take to decrease the likelihood of a breach in confidentiality. On the other hand, there are times when breaching confidentiality is necessary to protect patients. While specific regulations may differ slightly by region, typically health care providers must report to authorities when someone shares a desire to harm themselves or others. While the specific occasions when personal details will need to be shared are likely the same as in a traditional mental health facility, but when compiling organization policies, it may be worth reiterating. Specific to e-mental health is the determination of whether employees can have access off-site, work from home, or use personal devices. There are several benefits and drawbacks to allowing staff to access e-mental health services to help patients outside the office, and each organization will need to determine their comfort level with employees working remotely. Finally, an organizational policy should include the consequences for failing to meet the standards as outlined. Considering confidentiality and privacy concerns in an organizational policy is incredibly important, but especially for organizations in the e-mental healthcare field.

Specific types of e-mental health

E-mental health spans many different types of technology, each with specific benefits and drawbacks. Some options for e-mental health are websites, community chat groups, text messages, email with a medical professional, mobile apps and video chatting. Each has security concerns and the concerns must be balanced against the benefits each technology brings to a patient. Websites are available which provide mental health information for anyone who wants to access it, from anywhere in the world. While accessing online information has the fewest security concerns and little possibility for confidentiality breaches, the quality if information can vary and the information is not tailored to the patient. Websites can be a helpful tool and are the safest from a security perspective, but for many patients, treatment will be required in addition to tips learned online. A community chat group can be a good way to reach out for peer support where each person can learn from each other's perspectives. Ensuring privacy is largely dependent on the user refraining from sharing personal details. If a chat group assigns usernames rather than having users identified with their first or last names, extra privacy can be ensured. Chat groups which have guidelines laid out to ensure personal information is not shared can be a very safe option from a confidentiality standpoint. Group chat comes with the drawbacks of information being potentially shared which is not tailored to the needs of the user but is instead anecdotal and may not be accurate. Texting can be a type of e-mental health with either emergency hotlines which can be texted or medical professionals including text messaging into their follow up care. Often, text messages are not encrypted meaning there could be breaches in security or confidentiality and phone providers do not typically guarantee that text messages are completely secure ways of communicating. Texting has the benefits of immediate communication and answers to questions but is a time-consuming form of communication for the mental health professional. Email is another type of e-mental health platform as patients can email questions and receive answers from a professional without booking a face to face appointment. When used for simple, routine questions or clarification, email can be a great option, but like text messaging lacks some privacy guarantees. Email security varies, but having emails accessed by third parties who were not intended to receive the email is not uncommon. Mobile apps are a growing type of e-mental health. Apps can be used for many different purposes within e-mental health and each app has a different privacy policy. As each app is different, it is difficult to generalize how secure app-based e-mental health can be. It is best to check if conversations are encrypted and how much personal information is required from a patient before using an app for mental health help, advise or treatment. Finally, video chatting can be a good option for e-mental health treatment. Live online video chatting is typically a secure way for a patient to discuss concerns with a medical professional, as many video chatting websites and apps have security in place to protect against confidentiality breach. Additionally, if someone were to look through a patient's device, an email contents can be read, but a video discussion is not automatically recorded and saved. Video messages are a great option for people who live in remote areas and find attending face to face appointments a challenge. Video chatting is not without security risk but comes with most of the benefits of a face-to-face mental health appointment. Regardless of the type of e-mental health platform is utilized, keeping information private while using the internet is extremely important.

Ideas/ Tips

The Federal Trade Commission of the United States has published several tips for protecting personal information online (Federal Trade Commission, 2018). The first suggestion is to be alert to impersonators. While this applies to all online activity, it is advisable for a patient to research the e-mental health provider and attempt to determine their legitimacy. Additionally, just because an e-mental health provider is legitimate, people can impersonate companies by sending emails with links which can steal personal information from a computer or device. If an email is received, it is best to go to the company's website directly, rather than clicking on a link in an email. A good rule to go by is that the patient should initiate contact with a company. If a patient has not initiated contact, do not click on any emails and instead contact customer service directly as the email could be fraudulent. Additionally, it is important to safeguard personal information and have a level of awareness over what information may be required, and what should not be asked. If an e-mental health provider is requesting personal information like social insurance numbers, this is not appropriate, and the information may be used in fraudulent ways.

Encrypt Data

While encrypting data may sound complicated, an e-mental health patient can ensure their communication is encrypted without having a computer background or above average knowledge of technology. Encryption includes data being sent which is encoded so only the parties who are authorized to receive the information can view it. Encryption prevents sensitive information from being easily hacked. Before using an e-mental health service, look into the company's privacy policies which are likely available through their website, and see if encryption is included in their security plan. Some web browsers will include a "lock" icon next to the website address which also means the web browser considers the website safe to use. Before providing personal information, look for the lock icon.

Passwords

Passwords are extremely important when using the internet in general, but passwords are uniquely important when discussing e-mental health. Some of the content in e-mental health conversations can be extremely sensitive, and in some cases if family members read the details of conversations, the patient could be at risk. Having a strong password which is only known by the user is important to maintaining confidential conversations. A strong password is a password with six to ten characters, though ten is better, and a combination of lower and uppercase letters, numbers and symbols (Computer Hope, 2014). When choosing a password, some tips include choosing a phrase and taking the first letter from each word, or replacing numbers with words or letters. There are several methods for creating a secure password, the important part is to create something unique, but memorable for the user which isn't shared with anyone.

Information Sharing

Determining what information to share online, will depend on the type of technology being used, however it is best to speak in generalities and avoid divulging personal details where possible. Some websites, especially those featuring chat rooms, may request usernames be used as opposed to real names to protect the identity of users. When these protocols are in place, honor the restrictions and users should not share their names. While this is one example, it is a good habit to get into for a user to avoid sharing real names, specific locations, names of employers, etc. As explained previously, do not share social insurance numbers or banking information as there is unlikely a legitimate reason for a mental health provider to require such details.

For Organizations

The federal trade commission includes suggestions for protecting devices which can be helpful for healthcare providers attempting to add electronic therapy into their clinic. Consulting a knowledgeable information technologist, or IT professional who can assist with securing an office device for e-mental health uses. Using security software may seem like an obvious step for an office handling confidential information, or any internet user, but adding security software which directly addresses the security needs of the organization is incredibly important. An expert can assist with this process.

Training staff

Training staff in some basics in online security will be necessary if e-mental health is being added to a health care providers services, or a new business is attempting to work in e-mental health. The training can include local regulations, organization specific policies and general tips for maintaining client confidentiality. Ensuring staff know to avoid opening files or links emailed to them by unknown email addresses and avoiding public wi-fi when accessing work files are good tips for staff. Additionally, encouraging staff to keep devices in safe places and avoid using automatic login features will help prevent devices from being stolen and files accessed.

Barriers

Each organization will encounter unique barriers to introducing e-mental health into their practice. Specifically, when concerning the training of staff on security measures in an online space, one significant barrier is a lack of time. Workloads within healthcare in many areas of the world make allocating time to properly train staff difficult and expensive. While many can take for granted their safety and security while online, when a mental health professional enters an online space, the security of their patient must be considered and taken seriously. Rushed training can lead to a lack of compliance with policies by under trained staff. Taking the time to properly train staff can help patients' information be secure. While there are significant barriers to educating staff in security protocols, the time and cost invested will help create a professional e-mental health environment.

Conclusion

E-mental health creates an opportunity for both patients and medical professionals to utilize technology to help decrease the pain and difficulties which mental illness brings. While the benefits of e-mental health are numerous, there are drawbacks, including potential security and privacy issues which do not exist in traditional face-to-face mental health treatment. While each type of e-mental health platform will have different levels of risk, it is important to learn how best to protect personal information when bringing technology into mental health treatment. Patients and mental health professionals need to work together to find the best types of treatment available by weighing the benefits and drawbacks of each. Only then can the industry continue to grow and help reach more people with mental health struggles.

References

Computer Hope. (2018, November 26). What is a Password? Retrieved from https://www.computerhope.com/jargon/p/password.htm

Federal Trade Commission. (2018, November 2). How to Keep Your Personal Information Secure. Retrieved from https://www.consumer.ftc.gov/articles/0272-how-keep-your-personal-information-secure

Humphreys, K., Winzelberg, A., & Klaw, E. (2000). Psychologists' ethical responsibilities in Internet-based groups: Issues, strategies and a call for dialogue. Professional Psychology: Research and Practice, 39(2), 493-496.

McGrath, P., Wozney, L., Rathore, S.S., Notarianni, M., Schellenberg, M. (2018). Toolkit for e-Mental Health Implementation. Mental Health Commission of Canada. Ottawa, ON

8. Stigma and E-Mental Health

Introduction
When discussing mental health, stigma is an important topic to include. Stigma, or negative perceptions people have towards a specific group is a problem for mental health patients and causes a significant barrier to becoming well. Those with mental illnesses can be stigmatized anywhere, but law enforcement, healthcare professionals and those in their workplaces are consistently guilty of stigmatizing those with mental health issues. In addition, those within marginalized groups are at risk for further discrimination while trying to navigate the world with a mental illness. Being aware of stigmatization is one of several steps which everyone can take to reduce stigma for those with mental health issues, and is the first step to reducing stigmatization. E-mental health specifically can help those who suffer with mental illnesses by being an option which can be accessed from anywhere at any time. As a society, stigma is a significant problem and leads to discrimination and each individual needs to address the prejudices within themselves and work to replace stigma with empathy, understanding and compassion.

Definition of stigma
Stigma is a negative attitude of discredit which is

placed on a person by members of society based on the stigmatized individuals' attributes, lifestyle, medical situation or anything else about a person which makes them outcast. Stigma can apply to anyone, but those in minority groups are typically affected more by stigma. Stigmatized persons are looked down on by other people and are discriminated against. People who have experienced stigma, are feared and distrusted by people they encounter. This becomes particularly difficult when facing stigma from loved ones, employers or medical professionals. Stigma or even a fear or being stigmatized can lead to people being afraid of sharing with friends and family members, or fear of speaking honestly with medical professionals. Another aspect of stigma which is not always as obvious to people is self-stigmatization. When an individual encounters consistent negative attitudes from their community, people sometimes internalize these attitudes which leads to low self esteem and decreased quality of life. This chapter will specifically cover stigma and those suffering from mental health illnesses.

Causes of Stigma against those with mental illness

Stigma is a significant problem facing people with psychiatric disorders, but when considering the causes of stigma, the answer is not simple or straightforward. Dr. Marjorie Baldwin, in her book Beyond Schizophrenia: Living and Working with a Serious Mental Illness, outlines fives common causes of stigma and people with mental illnesses (Greenstein, 2016). The first cause Dr. Baldwin discusses is responsibility. People who struggle with mental illness can feel responsible for their thoughts, behaviors and attitudes, even when heavily impacted by the state of their mental health. Someone struggling with depression may feel lazy, for example, and feel responsible for their low mood. Comments from others asking someone to "snap out of it", only adds to the existing ideas that the person struggling is responsible for their illness. While there are many factors which can cause mental illness, the person who struggles with their mental health is not responsible. The next cause Dr. Baldwin discusses is stigma caused by uncertainty. In this case, uncertainty applies to the feeling of uncertainty when a person's mental health is unlikely to improve significantly. People can feel stigmatized when loved ones see their situation as hopeless. Similarly to a physical injury or disability, it may be difficult for loved ones to adjust to a new reality which includes a mental health diagnosis. This is especially true if a complex mental health diagnosis seems unlikely to improve over time or treatment. Along with uncertainty, which concerns the long term, another cause of stigma for people with mental illnesses is unpredictability, which focuses on the short term. People with mental health concerns may act differently than previously or act differently than people expect. Fidgeting and pacing are two examples of the symptoms which may be considered erratic by those who interact with the individual who has a mental illness. Unfortunately, unpredictability can lead to friends and loved ones pulling away and spending less time socially with someone perceived as unpredictable. Another cause of mental health stigma is incompetence. Viewing someone who has a mental illness as incompetent is an unfortunately common type of stigmatization, which assumes people are unable because of their diagnosis. This type of stigmatization can be seen in laws restricting the rights of people with mental illnesses, and in less obvious ways, like in the workplace. People hesitate to share their mental health diagnosis with coworkers out of a fear that the knowledge may limit future career advancement. This is an unfortunate reality that many people face, even though people with mental illness can hold a wide variety of jobs and contribute very positively to society. The final cause discussed by Dr. Baldwin is dangerousness. Fear of a mentally ill person reacting violently is an extension of a fear of unpredictability. While people struggling with mental health diagnosis can behave unpredictably, most people with mental illnesses are not violent and are more likely to be a victim of violence (National Alliance on Mental Illness, 2019). As a society, empathy and understanding needs to take the place of fear and stigmatization. People going through difficult times because of mental illness need positive support and a belief that recovery is possible. This belief needs to be echoed by their loved ones and community. We need to see people, not a diagnosis and end mental health stigma.

Stigma and Mental Health

Of the estimated 50 million Americans who live with a mental illness, less than half receive treatment for their condition. (Gluck, 2015) People who struggle under the weight of mental illness feel the need to hide their diagnosis from the people around them for fear of being stigmatized. Individuals fear stereotypes and negative attitudes associated with something they cannot control any more than an individual with a physical illness can. Media portrays people who struggle with mental illness as incompetent and prone to violence. This leads to a belief that those who suffer from mental illness are dangerous to be around. This is not accurate and people with mental illness are typically non-violent (Mental Health of America of Wisconsin, 2015). Along with portraying the mentally ill as violent, people who suffer from mental illness are often shown in the media as incompetent, leading to the idea that people with mental health issues are not suited to stressful careers or higher-level positions. Modern medical and psychological advancements have meant people receiving treatment for mental illness have a wide variety of careers and levels of responsibility in the workplace. A common misconception about mental illness is that those who suffer should be placed into specialized facilities to care for mental health issues. While institutions can be helpful for some, supports exist which enable people to live normal lives while under treatment for mental illness. These attitudes come from stigmatization and are frequently based on incorrect information and stereotypes perpetuated by the media.

Sites of Stigmatization

While stigma is something people carry with themselves as attitudes and beliefs, certain situations can showcase why stigma can be so problematic. Stigma can become especially obvious when dealing with law enforcement, healthcare professionals and those within their workplace. Each site of stigmatization can be navigated positively, but may require additional awareness.

Law Enforcement

For a person with a mental illness, dealing with law enforcement can be especially nerve wracking. Police are not consistently trained in interacting with those who have mental illnesses or in the prevention of stigmatizing behaviors. Each individual police department sets the training and the Mental Health Commission of Canada found the training to be non-existent in some regions, with multi-day tailored programs in other police departments (Coleman & Cotton, 2010). With such vastly different training in place, one step towards reduced stigmatization would be to include training for interacting with people with mental health issues into every police department. If law enforcement professionals are particularly upsetting due to a citizens mental state, a discussion with a therapist can help. Mental health professionals can help patients with strategies to cope through high stress situations, like dealing with law enforcement. As more and more police departments adopt comprehensive mental health training, the relationship between law enforcement and those with mental illnesses can change and hopefully, stigma by law enforcement can be reduced.

Healthcare

While stigma in healthcare is a complex subject, medical facilities can become a site of stigma for people with mental health issues and there are ways to improve the situation. Healthcare providers can actually be the cause of the deepest negative feelings of stigma, which may cause those with mental illnesses to postpone seeking care. (Langille, 2014) The Mental Health Commission of Canada (MHCC) has included "diagnostic overshadowing (wrongly attributing unrelated physical symptoms to mental illness), prognostic negativity (pessimism about chances for recovery) and marginalization (unwillingness to treat psychiatric symptoms in a medical setting)" (Langille, 2014) as concerning behaviors of health-care providers. In response, the MHCC has developed initiatives to reduce stigma within healthcare and evaluate existing programs in an attempt to better train healthcare professionals to identify and avoid stigmatizing language and behaviors when working with mentally ill patients. The programs have had positive results. Stigma in healthcare is a problem, but there are improvements happening in the industry and hopefully this will encourage more people to get the help they need and have less fear of stigma in healthcare facilities.

Workplace

Fear of stigma at work can be particularly complicated for a variety of reasons. People who struggle under the weight of mental illness may feel the need to hide symptoms while at work out of fear of discrimination. Each employment situation is different, and some corporate cultures are more open to giving employees time off to treat mental health issues. Other environments are less empathetic and may question if the person is in need of help. When discussing mental health with an employer, it can be helpful to know if mental health is addressed in company policies and benefits. Some employers include therapy in health insurance packages, and some include job protected time off for mental health treatment. Knowing what is included can help an employee feel more confident discussing mental illness with a supervisor. The Centre for Addiction and Mental Health recommends at least being clear with an employer about potential triggers or difficult aspects of work. The example The Centre for Addiction and Mental Health uses in their recommendations is if long meetings are difficult, notifying an employer that periodically leaving the room may be necessary (The Centre for Addiction and Mental Health, 2019). From an employer perspective, when an employee comes forward looking for assistance, being aware of the stigma which may exist and leading with understanding and empathy is the best way to help. Reinforcing that a mentally ill individual is not at fault for their condition and disclosing details about mental health takes courage may help an employee feel at ease and more likely to trust their employer in the future. As an employer, training staff to recognize mental illness as a relatively common type of illness and not a sign of weakness can help reduce stigma surrounding mental health in the workplace. Stigma surrounding mental health in the workplace unfortunately exists, but hopefully as a society steps can be taken to improve the conditions for those who struggle with mental health issues.

Combating stigma

There are several ways to combat mental health stigma. Education is an important tool which can help reduce stigma by removing the incorrect information people carry with themselves. The more people bravely speak about their mental health challenges and successes the more attitudes can shift on the topic and others can see that mental illness is nothing to feel shame for and ideally treatment should be as normalized as treatment for any physical illness. Take opportunities to share messages about mental health awareness on social media platforms to add another voice to the conversation. By posting about mental health issues, someone suffering can feel less alone and may be more likely to seek out help with mental health issues. Additionally, discussing mental health with family members is a great way to discover if there is a genetic history of mental illness within a family, and allowing any family members suffering with mental illnesses to know they have an ally. People can be moved to become educated when an issue affects someone they love, so openly discussing mental health issues can also lead to family members reaching out for information and reducing stigma through obtaining correct information. Knowing someone who has a mental illness can humanize mental illness sufferers and reduce the tendency to stereotype these individuals.

Pathstone Mental Health recommends seven strategies to reduce stigma (Pathstone, 2017). First, education and accurate information can help reduce stigma. Misinformation is a significant cause of stigma and discrimination. Second, being aware of how behaviors and attitudes can be affected by prejudices. While self-awareness is a difficult ability to obtain, anyone can adjust their attitudes if given a good reason. Be aware of the stereotypes which may exist and replace them by seeing someone as a well-rounded individual and not just their stereotypical traits. Next, avoid negative or derogatory language by choosing words used carefully. Stigmatized groups may request certain words no longer be used and everyone should attempt to avoid such potentially harmful language. The next recommended strategy to decrease stigma is to educate others. Respectfully challenging others when myths or stereotypes are presented can show people another side of an issue and help people who may stigmatize without realizing the potential harm. False ideas affect those who are stigmatized, so take opportunities when possible to pass on accurate, empathetic attitudes instead. Next, when discussing those who are discriminated against, focus on the positive, rather than the negative aspects of their lives. In the case of those who have mental health problems, their health is only one part of their overall person and people with such struggles can still make a positive impact on their communities. When given the chance, recognize the positive stories and share them when appropriate. The final recommendations for reducing stigmatization and discrimination are supporting people and including everyone. Support may look different for different people, but if a friend, family member or coworker is struggling with mental health issues, encourage treatment and their efforts to get help. Finally, including everyone applies to housing, employment and many other areas of a person's life. In Canada, laws against discrimination exist, and similar laws should be encouraged for everyone, so each human being has the same opportunities without discrimination or stigma. Reducing stigma is important for those who are stigmatized, and everyone needs to take part for real societal changes to be implemented.

Stigma and e-mental health treatment

When considering the impact stigma has on mental health treatment, some individuals are hesitant to seek treatment due to the perception associated with therapy and other treatment. While stigma can prevent someone from seeking treatment, e-mental health may be a method to reach those who are hesitant to go to a doctor or therapist. E-mental health includes tools to help with mental illness, integrated with technology. Some of the hurdles people face when looking for treatment options disappear when using e-mental health tools. For example, if someone is afraid to request a day off from work to visit a therapist, due to a fear of being stigmatized by their employer, chatting online with a counselor outside work hours can be an option which would eliminate the fear of stigma. Ideally, stigma within mental health treatment would eventually disappear and be looked at with the same understanding as physical health, but until society arrives at that point, e-mental health may be a great option. With apps, websites and chat options, among other e-mental health platforms, patients can reach out for help when it is needed, in the moment and hopefully with less stigma attached to reaching out. Additionally, some e-mental health websites are modelled as peer support with trained volunteers who refer patients to professionals when needed. This type of peer support is a type of e-mental health but may not carry the same stigma for someone as making an appointment with a doctor or therapist. As e-mental health grows in scope and popularity, more and more people will be able to reach services from their homes, or wherever help may be needed and can do so privately and ideally, without stigma.

Navigating social climates

A social climate is a term used by sociologists to discuss the attitudes and feelings a group have on a certain subject. Social climate can be influenced by several factors, like political climate, social issues, and media presentations. These dominant beliefs held by the population can lead to important conversations which may have been considered taboo previously. The "#metoo" movement was started by women who wanted to start a conversation about sexual assault. As the movement grew, stigma around discussing sexual harassment and assault lessened and people who were untouched by the issue were able to see how common sexual assault actually is. The "#metoo" movement become viral because celebrities and influencers with large social media followings used their platforms to spread the message. Stigma was positively affected and while not perfect, the climate changed for victims. Mental health has had a similar shift over the past as more and more people speak openly about how common mental health issues are. As more and more people use their platforms to shift the social climate towards mental health into an open and understanding space, stigma will also be reduced and people with mental illness will be able to interact with people with less fear of stigmatization and discrimination.

Heightened stigma in specific disadvantaged groups

Some individuals find themselves in the unfortunate reality where they are stigmatized for both their mental illness and another aspect of their lives. These individuals are especially at a disadvantage when navigating workplaces, healthcare or interactions with law enforcement. Individuals who have experienced stigma and discrimination due to race, gender, lifestyle or any number of factors may hesitate to seek mental health help because they have been stigmatized before. This adds extra responsibility to those who interact with someone in this situation to avoid stigmatizing language and create a safe environment for the individual. Everyone needs to work to avoid stigmatizing language and behavior, but when interacting with those who experience stigma in more than one area of their lives, even more care and empathy is needed.

Conclusion

Stigma and discrimination are important problems which affect everyone. The best way to fight stigmatization is with education. By learning about the challenges and abilities which others have, people can be viewed as more than a stereotype, and instead a well-rounded individual. While stigma can happen everywhere, law enforcement, medical professionals and employers can cause the most harm through stigmatization and must pay attention to reducing stigmatizing language and behavior. E-mental health can help with mental health treatment by reaching people who may be reluctant to seek mental health treatment because of stigma. Everyone can improve the stigma which impacts those with mental illness every day.

References

Centre for Addiction and Mental Health. (2019). Mental Health, Stigma and the Workplace. Retrieved from https://www.camh.ca/en/camh-news-and-stories/mental-health-stigma-and-the-workplace

Coleman, T. G., & Cotton, D. (2010). Police Interactions with Persons with a Mental Illness: Police Learning in the Environment of Contemporary Policing. Police Interactions with Persons with a Mental Illness: Police Learning in the Environment of Contemporary Policing. Mental Health and the Law Advisory Committee. Retrieved from https://www.mentalhealthcommission.ca/sites/default/files/Law_Police_Interactions_Mental_Illness_Report_ENG_0_1.pdf

Gluck, S. (2015, January 15). Stigma and Discrimination: The Effect of Stigma, HealthyPlace. Retrieved on 2019, September 3 from https://www.healthyplace.com/stigma/stand-up-for-mental-health/stigma-and-discrimination-the-effect-of-stigma

Greenstein, L. (2016, December 28). Understanding What Causes Stigma. Retrieved from https://www.nami.org/Blogs/NAMI-Blog/December-2016/Understanding-What-Causes-Stigma

Langille, J. (2014, January 24). Reducing stigma in health-care settings. Retrieved from https://www.canadian-nurse.com/en/articles/issues/2014/january-2014/reducing-stigma-in-health-care-settings

Mental Health of America of Wisconsin. (2015). Stigma: Building Awareness & Understanding. Retrieved from http://www.mhawisconsin.org/Data/Sites/1/media/fact-sheets-2015/stigma-building-awareness-and-understanding-2015.pdf

National Alliance on Mental Illness. (2019). Violence and Gun Reporting Laws. Retrieved from https://www.nami.org/learn-more/mental-health-public-policy/violence-and-gun-reporting-laws

Pathstone Mental Health. (2017). Seven Important things we can do to reduce Stigma and Discrimination. Retrieved from https://www.mendthemind.ca/stigma/seven-important-things-we-can-do-reduce-stigma-and-discrimination/

9. Kids & mobile apps

The cost/benefit yield of information technology can be unapologetically double-sided. The information age has imbued speed, power, and capability into our most critical social and economic institutions. However, detriments like human over-reliance and personal data vulnerabilities beget public skepticism around how, and to what extent info-tech is utilized in societies (see; bank data breaches - also see; level 1 trauma centre during a power-outage)

Psychiatry has experienced no shortage of advancements in information technology. To practitioners, innovations in this field often represent a revolution in workflow. Computational methods help streamline diagnosis and treatment, remote therapy solutions mend care-access disparities, while other modern tools help ameliorate mental-health-care processes.

Until the last decade (2010-2020) mental-health information technology seldom catered to consumer-based usage models. Advancement efforts in this area were most-often dedicated to improving efficiencies for practitioners and officers of mental-health care. With information technology now perforating client-practitioner care access models, mental health institutions took notice of shortfalls in technology utilization for patient self-care.

Development of the first e-mental health tools for public use began as early as 1999. From a user's experience, these platforms were often cumbersome - relying on 'early' incantations of computing and internet that were unable to fully optimize a user's experience - thus, pushing e-mental health toward the category of 'fringe' and 'boutique' research. Until computation and network efficiency could contend with user-preferences, accessibility issues continued to stifle successful adoption of e-mental health tools, keeping them obsolete, out of sight, and out of mind to the general public. However, with the explosion of 'next-gen' mobile technology such as smartphones and advanced mobile networking in the late 2000's, e-mental health took an unexpected leap into its new chariot; mobile apps.

With mobile app development becoming more affordable and captivating for users, proprietors of e-mental health discovered a gateway to bolstering mental-health for children and youth through applications compatible with their smartphones.

Children and youth inhabit a particularly daunting demographic in terms of engagement and accessibility regarding the uptake of healthcare education, resources, and patient self-care. When soliciting the attention and patronage of children and youth, health-care practitioners must contend with demographic-exclusive dynamics in order to fully access and leverage young people's attention. With careful consideration of tone, style, colloquialisms and popular-culture, it is possible to craft products and communications material capable of honing the consideration of young people. However, therein lies a fundamental problem for e-mental health's proprietors; healthcare institutions are not inherently competitive marketers. What's more, mercantilistic app and entertainment developers understand the finite nature of youth attention, and prioritize out-advertising other competitors eager to capture the attention of young people.

How is one to contend with dominant market forces despite the potential public good of an e-health product? While there may be no clear-cut answer to this quagmire, it is worth considering that healthcare is part of a broad social-infrastructure that is particularly effective in procuring and coordinating resources for a common goal. In the case of Canadian e-mental health, several provinces have announced public-health coordination efforts between regional hospitals, schools, and social services to fight mental health stigma and service discontinuity. After the rollouts of recent initiatives in 2012 and 2018, Albertan investigators saw a sharp rise in utilization of smartphone e-mental health apps, online psychotherapy, peer-support, and other internet-enabled e-health tools in demographics most likely to engage with public institutions. The most frequently and consistently engaged demographic, in these cases, was children and youth.

International statistics currently indicate that e-mental health is gaining popularity world-wide among young people. This may be due in-part to optimizations in communications and advertising strategies, the already-present likelihood of younger people engaging with info-tech, or the coordinated efforts of public institutions that serve youth to encourage engagement with mental health care tools and resources. At this time, there is scant research about how youth established such a large stake in the usership of e-mental health, and why the trend transpired in the first place. The matter may be of little consequence to clinicians, pathologists, and frontline-health professionals; youth are using e-mental health apps, and despite research interest in this area being fairly new, preliminary results from several studies show prognostic outcomes of children and youth who use e-mental health apps are positive. Regardless, the 'why' is still shrouded - the consequences of which inevitably stifle further optimization of access points for youth mental health care, particularly in the e-health space.

    Unsurprisingly, Millennials (people born between the years 1980 and 2000) create the largest user base among those who utilize e-mental health apps. This is unsurprising because of contiguity between the generation's coming-of-age and propagation of capable computing technology. However, this collision of generation and technology raises contextual questions about whether or not Millenial's adoption of e-mental health was due to time-and-place, or if social factors, perhaps technology itself, precipitated mental health issues in this population - creating demand for accessible, affordable mental-health care in the form of e-mental health.

    Millennial culture is sometimes considered by sociologists to be a 'black-box'. Rapid advancement and integration of information and communication technologies propagated what was considered a seamless and instantaneous connection between people - novel and distinct to that of face-to-face contact. How did this global communications overhaul affect millennials culturally and developmentally? Of course, this technological revolution represented fertile ground for investment, giving rise to social-media corporations whose business model relies on constant user engagement and data collection for advertising and monetization. The question remains; what mental health outcomes have millennials lost or gained as a result of a sudden corporate interest in their information and the enticing social media platforms that procure it?

    This text is not intended to be an anthology on social-media, millennials, the internet, or the determinants of mental-health that lie therein. However, the advent of powerful infotainment communicators raises potent questions about the relationship between their use and the mental-health impacts bestowed upon millennial users. An all-to-familiar paradox arises; which came first - the chicken or the egg? That is, did the rapid creation and integration of online communications inadvertently propagate a system of social-credit, serving to perpetually invalidate youth and degrade their mental-health? Or, were issues of mental health already present in the population - allowing e-technologies such as social media to catalyze communion among sufferers with compatible experience? At this moment, the jury is largely out. Despite this, various disciplines of medicine and social science have published scathing works illustrating social-media and info-tech dependence as detrimental intoxicants to the health and development of young people. Needless to say, social media apps are not considered to be e-mental health tools.

Conclusion

Evaluation of the shift to e-mental health is a complex task and requires us to go beyond merely considering the virtual counselling taking place. The larger environmental context is a landscape littered by unique socio-cultural, legislative, and historical elements. While changing these features to improve services on the ground might not be feasible or timely, these system-level aspects will need to be addressed for successful longer-term implementation of e-mental health services given certain stresses. Perhaps the biggest stress currently is the COVID-19 pandemic that wreaks havoc as we write this piece, it is forcing our systems of governance and healthcare to rethink conventional delivery of mental health care.

Nevertheless, there are considerations and pitfalls that should be top-of-mind. These include being steadfast about listening to and upholding guidance from public health associations, being skeptical of misinformation online, and the traps of cyber-abuse. Privacy considerations go hand-in-hand with digitizing information and government policies relating to reimbursement of services provided virtually and for service coordination for clients particularly in remote areas (insufficient access to reliable internet services) with complex needs are still issues that require further development of infrastructure. Linguistics and communication methods should also kept in mind when tailoring e-mental health technology to a layman audience and people who may struggle with being able to appositely use what they are provided with.